The Dill Pickle and Green Olive Diet and Exercise Plan

The Dill Pickle and Green Olive Diet and Exercise Plan

K. S. Faulkner

iUniverse, Inc.

New York Lincoln Shanghai

The Dill Pickle and Green Olive Diet and Exercise Plan

iUniverse books may be ordered through booksellers or by contacting:

iUniverse
2021 Pine Lake Road, Suite 100
Lincoln, NE 68512
www.iuniverse.com
1-800-Authors (1-800-288-4677)

Because of the dynamic nature of the Internet, any Web addresses or links contained in this book may have changed since publication and may no longer be valid.

You should not undertake any diet/exercise regimen recommended in this book before consulting your personal physician. Neither the author nor the publisher shall be responsible or liable for any loss or damage allegedly arising as a consequence of your use or application of any information or suggestions contained in this book.

ISBN: 978-0-595-48459-1 (pbk)
ISBN: 978-0-595-60552-1 (ebk)

Printed in the United States of America

Contents

Introduction

I think I have tried most of the popular fad diets. I have eaten boiled eggs for breakfast lunch and dinner, I have consumed only protein for all meals, I have done the grapefruit, the water and the cabbage diets, I have done the Atkins, Weight Watchers, and the Kaiser diets.

I have been a member of as many as three health clubs at the same time. I have been a member of Gyms such as Golds, 24 Hour Fitness, Right Stuff, Curves and a number of small single club entities.

I have purchased 2 tread mills, one elliptical trainer, a Health Rider, the Gazelle, a stepper, a ski machine, 2 rowing machines, some strange machines that were subsequently sold shortly after purchase, 2 weight cages, and a universal weight machine.

I have even tried some really strange approaches such as the rubber suits that you connect to your vacuum cleaner while you do housework that is supposed to reduce inches from the covered parts of your body with only one use. I guess that this is supposed to make you sweat and therefore reduce the liquids that you are retaining. I know it was so uncomfortable that I could only stand wearing it for a few minutes and when I removed the garment (if you can call it that) my under-garments were saturated with sweat.

I have also tried the Ab Roller, the Ab Lounge and a lot of other really strange looking equipment that I forget the names of. I have tried the monster rubber bands for resistance. I have worn ankle weights while I do housework and you can still find various sized of dumbbells through out my house.

I am not saying this because weight loss is hopeless. I am just saying that, unless you are really committed, weight loss that involves doing something that you do not enjoy is difficult.

Have I learned anything?

- I have learned that if a diet or eating program is not satisfying, it will be abandoned.

- I have learned that if an exercise is not fun I will not continue with it past a week or so.

- I have learned that just owning exercise equipment does nothing more than clutter up the house.

- Exercise equipment make very expensive clothes hangers.

- I can exercise for hours if I am enjoying what I am doing but I am bored after about 5 minutes if I am not enjoying what I am doing.

- If I tell myself that I am on a diet then I am hungry all of the time

- When I am not on a diet I can even miss meals when I am busy doing things that I like without feeling that I am starving to death.

- When I am on a diet I crave really bad foods.

- I gain weight back a lot faster than I lose it

- I usually gain back more than I lost in the first place.

Does any of the above sound familiar?
What is the solution?

- A custom diet and exercise program developed just for me by me

- A custom diet and exercise program developed just for you by you

No one knows what I will enjoy doing and eating more than I do.
No one knows what you will enjoy doing and eating more than you do.
Consequently, I am the best person to develop a diet and exercise plan that I can stick with and will work for me and you are the best person to develop a diet and exercise plan that you can stick with and will work for you.
From here on out I will chronicle my quest to establish the perfect diet and exercise program for me. I have included pages at the end of the book for your diet and exercise program development.

◆   ◆   ◆

I wanted a program that I could stick with without feeling deprived. I also needed a program that would work. If I was unsuccessful I would need to buy yet another complete wardrobe, which has always proven to be very expensive, and I would need to find more storage space for my old clothes, I have always intended to be able to fit back into these smaller sizes, I currently have a second home that I use solely for storage.

The first task on my list was to find a mid meal snack to substitute for the potato chips, hot dogs and chocolate bars that I crave any time I pursue a diet program. I have found that when I am not on a diet, I do not have these cravings as much.

OK, so I went to a store and walked up and down the isles looking for foods that I like and then reading the labels. I was looking for 4 things. Serving sizes that I could observe without a problem, calorie count, fat content (good or bad), and sugar content. I do not have a problem with salt, otherwise my ultimate choices would have been problematic.

One comment on serving sizes: When I am on a diet, serving sizes are pretty much the whole box or bag. If one serving is 100 calories but that is only one cookie and the box contains 20 cookies then if it is in my cupboard I will eat the entire box in one sitting making the calories per serving when I am eating them to be equal 2000. The same thing goes for cereal once you start planning your meals.

If you are the type of person that likes to cut to the chase and you are already getting bored reading this book after less than 10 pages, then you should skip to the back of the book and go shopping for midday or midnight snacks that will satisfy you enough to wait for any more food until a real meal is called for. Sometimes any progress at all is enough to help you focus. Most of the diet and exercise books that I have read in the past gave me the feeling that I needed to finish the book before I started the plan.

I might mention that I have such a short attention span that I very seldom ever finished the books and I never started the plans. The only diet and exercise plans that I have ever started and stuck with were in the 2-3 maximum page range or easy reading with lots of pictures.

Observations

I think it is unfair that I can merely think about eating and I gain weight but I cannot lose weight by thinking about exercise. I can't even lose weight by buying exercise equipment or by joining a gym.

Who do they think they are kidding when they label short fat clothes as Petite? There is nothing Petite about a size 24. They should be arrested for false advertising. The label should be SW for short and wide. And what is this 1X, 2X and 3X. Do we need a whole new numbering scheme once we progress above a size18?

You have to be a detective to find the "WOMEN'S" department in some of the nicer clothing stores. The clothes that they put out front where everyone can find them only fit a fashion model on a diet or her anorexic twin sister. The larger sizes are hidden in the basement or someplace upstairs. Are they trying to make us exercise to find our department? Don't they know we will just take the elevator? How much more electricity do you think it takes to have the elevator lifting our weight rather than that size ZERO super model?

Serving size denotations are a joke too. A serving size is the entire container, however large it is, because that is how much I am going to eat in one sitting once I start eating. I hate looking at the back that says calories per serving 140 but servings per container 14. I then have to multiply calories by servings per container to figure out how much I just ate (Not Fair).

Even if I don't eat the entire container, because I feel guilty, I usually only leave one or two servings. Then I have to take the number of servings, subtract what I left in the container and then multiply by calories per serving. This is way above the amount of brain power that I want to use just to eat a snack.

I also think that the bathroom scales that you buy for your home are a joke. If you are one of those people who really need to weigh themselves, your weight won't even register on these pathetically inept pieces of equipment. You still have to go to the doctor to find out how much you weigh.

Or maybe this is a good thing. If the bathroom scales won't go any higher then I guess that is how much I weigh. It is the same sort of logic when you are speeding and the needle to the speedometer is bouncing up and down on the number at the far right of the gauge and you think that you are only going 115 miles per hour. Works for me!!

I know that there are all sorts of pills out there that promise to take the weight off. I also know from watching others who took new medications to help with their weight in the past that some of them can cause more problems than they cure. I have always been too afraid to take these new drugs until they have been very well tested over time. So I guess I am stuck with the old fashion methods of weight reduction.

OK, enough of my complaints about the unfairness of our individual metabolisms. What can we do about it without declaring that we are on a diet and that we are going to start exercising? By the way, this sort of declaration, even if it is only to your dog, will doom you to failure. It may even send you into some sort of feeding frenzy. For me, the mere mention of the word diet makes me really hungry and the thought of exercise makes me want to take a long nap.

Food Selection Rules

I know it sounds easy, but if it was that easy why do I keep gaining weight.

Rule #1

Never, Never, Never go food shopping when you are HUNGRY.

When I shop, the food knows when I am hungry. I walk up and down the isles and the Oreo cookies, Breyer's Ice Cream and Chocolate bars jump right into my shopping cart when I am not looking and I don't realize they are there until I reach the checkout stand. Of course I feel bad if the clerks are forced to return the treats to their original homes so I take them home, or worse yet I may eat them on the way home, hoping to dispose of any evidence of my binge before entering the house.

If you find your stomach growling while you are shopping for food you have 3 choices to try to stay on track.

1. Go home and eat, coming back only after you are no longer hungry.

2. Buy a healthy snack, go to the car to eat it and return when you are no longer hungry

3. Use one of those carry baskets for your groceries, try to stick to buying what you need. At least a carry basket full of bad foods is not as damaging as a full cart of them and you can develop your arm muscles carrying the food that you select.

Rule #2

If possible, avoid the isles in the store that cause you the most problems.

Those isles may be the frozen food, bread, candy or cookie isles. I also know that the store employees and owners are part of the conspiracy against us when they place candy close to the checkout stand and ice cream across from the frozen vegetables.

An occasional slip is to be tolerated. Also, just because you buy the food doesn't mean that you have to eat it. You may even know some skinny friend that you can give it to.

Rule #3

Don't keep bad foods in your house, car or at work.

You will not be as tempted to break your diet if the food available where you live, work and play is healthy, low in calories and appealing.

Sometimes I hear the argument from parents (mothers in particular) that they do not want to deprive their family while they are on the diet so they have to have cookies, candy and ice cream in the house. My answer is simple: Cookies, candy and ice cream are not good for your children or your husband. While your significant others may not have weight problems now, eating enough of those high calorie foods may cause them to have a weight problem in the future. In addition, having these foods readily available at home encourages unhealthy eating habits to form even if they don't cause weight gain. Try making healthy snacks available and you may avoid health problems for them in the future.

In addition to being unattractive excess weight can lead to other health problems for our loved ones in the future. Do yourself and your family a favor by leaving the unhealthy foods in the store to tempt the super models and learn to keep healthy snacks at home for yourself and family members.

Foods that we should stay away from will show up enough other places where we have no control such as parties, meetings, and family dinners. Keeping these foods in places that we have control over is adding insult to injury by deliberately sabotaging our progress.

Rule #4

When you shop make a list and stick to it

I have yet to actually put potato chips, cheese cake, chocolate bars, ice cream and candy on a grocery list unless I am having guests over for snacks. Guess what ends up in my shopping basket when I do not have a shopping list.

One of the benefits of picking menus for the coming week is that you know what you need to buy. When making out the menu you can check the needed ingredients against those that you have in the house and add any missing ingredients to your shopping list. In the absence of a shopping list you are more likely to walk up and down all of the isles looking for the food on the shelves to jog you memory as something that you need.

In the absence of a shopping list you are more likely to buy foods that you should not be eating and you are less likely to remember all of the ingredients that you need for your chosen menus. You will need to go to the store more frequently, thus adding unneeded temptation for the additional trips. In addition to helping with your diet a shopping list can help with transportation expenses because you get all of your needed items in one shopping trip and forgo the need to return to the store for items that you forgot without a list.

Another trick that helps a lot, since when you diet you are more tempted by the bad things that are not on your list, is to make the list and get someone else to do the shopping for you. This only works if the other person is health conscious and can resist the bad treats that you are trying to avoid. I am lucky and I have someone that is very good about shopping for only good, healthy and low calorie foods. I also would never put bad stuff on the list if I was going to have him do the shopping, as it would be admitting that I am eating those items. My grocery list is much more likely to be healthy if I am getting him to do the shopping for me.

Rule #5

Never allow yourself to accept failure

So many people are doomed before they ever really start a diet and exercise program. I know, I used to be one of them. It seemed that every time I started to think about taking control of my eating the urge to binge would hit me. I could be 5-10 minutes into my diet and I would feel like a failure as I dipped into my large bowl of ice cream or worse yet as I ate spoonful after spoonful of cookie dough without any intentions of baking any cookies.

Dieting makes me hungry. Even if I have just consumed my normal meal just the thought of the diet makes me feel like eating everything in sight.

If you can resist the urge to binge it is a good thing. If you cannot resist the urge and you are staring at the empty bowl that originally contained 3 scoops of triple calorie chocolate ice cream in front of you, please do not feel like a failure. This is just a little detour off of your health quest.

I know that this is hard. In the past when I would binge, feel like a failure and drop the diet idea I would usually binge for days. Sulk for weeks and eventually return to the task of getting healthy again but only after gaining another 5–10 pounds. The trick is to try to break this cycle.

Rule #6

Make every calorie count

I can have 4 egg whites and one yolk and the calories in this meal will be less than if I had 2 whole eggs. I can have 2 slices of dry toast and the calorie content is less than when I have one slice of buttered toast (of course I use a lot of butter). One of my favorite dieting meals is an over medium 4 white one yolk egg dish as a sandwich between 2 dry slices of toast. I use salt and pepper to taste and may even add a very thin slice of onion for more flavor.

If I were to make deviled eggs and add onions, celery, capers, water chestnuts and pickles to replace ¾ of the egg yolks the resulting food would have a lot more taste and a lot less calories. Another of my favorite meals is chicken salad. I use very little mayonnaise and I add water chestnuts, onions, black pepper and sometimes cucumbers. These additional ingredients make the chicken go a lot further as a meal and they lower the calorie content per serving. I dice all of the additional items very small and the salad is great as a stuffing for tomatoes or you can just put in the center of a bed of brown rice.

I am sure that you can think of a lot of substitutions that will lower the calorie content of your favorite foods.

Food Selection—The Quest for Snacks

This is the first part of the book where you will need the work pages from the back of your book. The outcome from this exercise should be snacks and treats that are quick, easy and will not ruin your diet.

Your mission, should you choose to accept it, is to travel to your favorite grocery store with the task of buying only snacks for between meals and midnight awakenings.

Before you leave to go food shopping remember Rule # 1 and eat something healthy so that you are not shopping hungry.

The snacks should be small, satisfying and out of the ordinary. They should require no preparation. They should truly make you feel that you have devoured a treat. These treats should be low in calories and fat if possible. Think it is impossible. Well, maybe, but you might be surprised.

You will have your best results if you start at one end of the store go up and down all of the isles and end at the opposite end of the store. Check out everything that sounds good. By the time you are done you will have a better idea of what has been causing you trouble in past diets and also what sort of calorie content to expect from different types of foods.

Use the work pages to itemize the foods that sound good keeping track of the calorie, fat and sugar content. Once you have filled out the work pages you will use these pages to fill out the Snack Selection Final List that you can use when you create your shopping lists and menu guides.

If going to the store simply to make a list of treats seems like a waste of time and gas you can always get one of those calorie guides to foods and go through the book to find snacks that you feel will be satisfying. Make sure that your book also has fat and sugar content. This type of book is good too because you can compare the products from different companies to see which is the best for your diet. It is a lot easier to compare items when they are listed together than it is to compare the packages in the store. Regardless of which method you use the result should be that you find satisfying snack choices that will keep you from feeling deprived on the diet that you are designing for yourself.

I found that my favorite treats that met all of these rules were Dill Pickles and Green Olives. I also purchased some raw nuts, dried fruit, and a can of unsweetened pie cherries the cherries were one of my favorites as a child.

I have yet to wake up in the middle of the night with a craving for puffed rice cakes or celery. If that is what you come home from the store with, then I think you are fooling yourself and I don't think that you really tried.

One of my favorite snacks is homemade trail mix. I don't like peanuts, so most store bought trail mixes don't work for me. My homemade trail mixes have been known to have only 2 ingredients at times (walnuts and sweeten dried cranberries). I also like dried sour cherries and cashews. These trail mixes, while very satisfying are not low calorie, so package them in small lots and try to behave your self instead of opening and eating all of your packages in one sitting.

I have also found some very satisfying low calorie yogurt, pudding and jerky. Nabisco is producing new boxes of 100 calorie snacks. These are individually packaged snacks such as cookies or chips that taste amazingly like the original but contain only 100 calories per package. The only problem that I have with these snacks is that I find myself opening more than one package when I am really hungry which means that the calorie content of my snack is double or triple what it should be.

Don't let bold letters on the front of the package lure you into purchasing foods that will sabotage your diet. While Nonfat sounds like it should be good it does not mean that it is low in calories. It could be loaded with sugar. Same for Sugar free, it sounds good but it does not mean that the food is Fat free or even low fat. Be sure to look at the back to find out what the real fat and sugar content are, as well as the sodium content and any other ingredient that you may be allergic or sensitive to.

Also pay attention to the servings per package and decide if you can live by those numbers. If not then figure out how many servings you would make the package stretch for. Even a small Craker Jack bag has 3.5 servings per container at 120 calories per serving. That means in my house that same package contains only one serving and the calories per serving are 420. Doesn't sound as good as 120 calories but it is realistic based on my eating habits.

Potato chip packages are some of the worst. Even the calories per serving sound pretty bad and then you read on to find that the bag contains more than one serving. How unfair because there is no way that I am going to save any for another serving especially if it is my favorite of Salt and Vinegar potato chips.

I know it is not fair to ask you to pick healthy snacks, so I won't. But if you find some healthy snacks that end up on your list because you like them you might want to give them a higher priority when selecting a snack when you are hungry. For example, my snack list has the following items on it:

- Olives

- Dill pickles

- Unsweetened Tart Cherries

- Nabisco 100 calorie snack packs

- Bing Cherries

- Grapes

- Tapioca Pudding

- Cashews

- Almonds

- Dried Peaches

- Yogurt

When ever possible I try to go for the fresh fruit and yogurt for snacks.

In the middle of the night, however, I find that olives are about the only food on my list that is both quick and satisfying. I simply have to go to the refrigerator, open the olive jar, remove one or two olives, pop them in my mouth, chew, swallow and return to bed. I can't remember ever waking a second time and feeling hungry after this little snack. Some of my favorite olives are those stuffed with jalapeños or garlic. I like spicy food so these satisfy two cravings at once. I recently purchased a jar of olives where the serving size was 1.5 olives. Yep in the middle of the night when I get up for my snack I will be sawing one of the olives in half so that I can obey the serving size. So if 1.5 olives is a serving and that serving has 10 calories then when I eat 2 it will be **13.3333333** calories or better about thirteen and a half calories. Maybe they expected these to be sliced on pizza.

Food Selection—Meals

If you live alone or you just eat alone, your meal selection process is much easier than if you are responsible for the food purchase and preparation for others.

As with shopping for snacks.... Never go shopping for food if you are hungry.

I would also add that it helps if you eat a low calorie snack prior to starting your food prep for meals. If you cook while hungry, any bad snacks in the refrigerator have a tendency to fly into your mouth whenever you open the door to get ingredients for your meal. Another hazard of cooking while really hungry is that you eat most of the meal before you finish cooking and there is nothing (or very little) left for your family to eat once it is done.

I remember from years gone by when my sister and I used to make tollhouse cookies on the weekends. We ate so much of the dough that we only actually baked about $1/10^{th}$ of the batch that we had prepared. We started making a double batch so that there would be a decent quantity of baked cookies to show for our efforts. The problem was that we liked the dough better than the finished cookies. In the end we decided to just make the dough and freeze it for consumption uncooked and we skipped the baking step. (I might add that this cut our prep time from start to finish by a lot by skipping the preheating and baking steps.). We were actually able to consume less of the dough in the process because we knew it would be in the freezer later if we had another craving.

OK.... If you prepare your meals separately from others then there are a number of prepackaged low calorie meals available in the frozen food section. Be sure to note the calorie and fat content but most of the meals that you should be eating will have those items clearly displayed on the front of the package and may also include such words as Lean, Low Calorie and Healthy.

Remember that Salads, while low in calories without dressing, may rival the calorie count of a Big Mac once you add the dressing. If you love salads, as I do, you could try purchasing salad dressing mixes and just mix them with less of the fat. I use Good Seasons Italian dressing mix as a salad dressing and as a marinade for meat.

One of my favorite lunches is a breadless sandwich. I take lunchmeat and wrap it around a pickle, a pepper or an onion and eat it like a burrito. Sometimes I will take a lettuce leaf and put my sandwich ingredients on it instead of using bread.

Be creative when you fix your meals. One thing that dooms many diets is boredom. If you keep your meals interesting, you will be less likely to stray.

Be sure to pay attention to each meal. If you plan really good healthy low calorie dinners but eat a Big Mac for lunch and have Eggs Benedict for breakfast you may not achieve your weight loss goals.

You may want to break up the food selection for meals into 3 processes. I have always found that when one single process is overwhelming that breaking it into multiple less complicated steps helps. You could do your food research for breakfast, then for lunch and finally for dinner separately. Or you could do them separately and in a different order. What ever feels best to you will work. After all this is your diet and exercise book, written for you by you.

Breakfast selections

One popular selection for breakfast is cereal. Please read the serving sizes for this. The cereal box may claim to be the best diet food since grapefruit but if the serving size is a half cup and the only satisfying quantity is two cups then you need to multiply the calories per serving by four.

Try different healthy cereals to see if you like any of them. Pay close attention to sugar content when buying cereals. If the cereal has nuts in it you will need to watch the fat content as well.

Plain oatmeal is always a possibility. You can add fresh fruit and cinnamon for sweetness.

Eggs are another popular breakfast selection. Just know that the yolk is not low calorie. If eggs are on your menu you might try one yolk with four egg whites. This combination will have less calories then two eggs and should be as satisfying.

If you like pancakes try using whole grain mixes and make them from scratch. If you like French toast then try the one yolk to four whites in this recipe too. For syrup you can puree fresh fruit and add some low calorie yogurt. Get creative.

Lunch selection

Lunch is a good time for soup or sandwiches. As mentioned earlier, sandwiches don't have to contain bread. You could use lettuce leaves or lunchmeat for the outer layer of a wrap. You can also find some healthy diet breads that will not destroy your diet.

There are many healthy soups too. Pay attention to the serving size and watch the sodium content if you have problems with salt.

I like making meat salads (beef, chicken or tuna) with high quantities of roughage such as water chestnuts, cucumber and onions. This can then be used to stuff a tomato, a whole wheat pita, lettuce leaf or if you must insist bread.

Dinner selection

Select foods that you like. If you eat alone there are a lot of healthy, low calorie frozen single serving meals that are available. I think the prepackaged food idea is why one of the popular diet programs works so well. People tend to eat convenient foods. Why else would the fast food restaurants be so popular?

One of the problems that I have with the prepackaged foods is that I get hungry while I wait for the food to cook and I snack even while my healthy meal is cooking. Even if it only takes five minutes of cooking time I will be snacking during that time. I will even snack while I wait for the cooked food to cool enough to eat.

I solve this problem by putting the food in to cook and return to what ever I was doing after setting a timer so that I know when the food will be done. Once the food is out of the oven or microwave I again set the timer and return to what I was doing while I wait for the food to cool. As long as I am not in the kitchen and I occupy my time I can avoid snacking and can stick to the food that I have on my menu for that meal.

If you are going to prepare your own meals, watch the serving sizes for carbohydrates and your meats. If you like high calorie vegetables you will have to watch the serving sizes for these too.

Try to stick with lean cuts of meat. The white meat of the chicken and turkey are leaner than the dark meat. Make sure if you are eating chicken or turkey that you skip eating the skin, this has more calories than any other part of the bird. If you like Kentucky Fried Chicken you may find that it is much less tasty without the skin but it will be much less fattening if you remove it. A round steak is a leaner cut of meat than a T-bone steak or a Filet. A stir-fry can turn a number of boring ingredients into something interesting.

A note about recipes: Many recipes sound interesting but contain unhealthy ingredients. I don't let that stop me. I make all sorts of substitutions and come out with some awesome meals. I substitute olive oil for butter in most recipes, I substitute canola oil mayonnaise for the regular version, I substitute whole wheat flour for white flour, I substitute whole wheat pasta and brown rice for their more processed cousins. If I want to use a recipe I will find a substitute for any bad ingredients.

Go Shopping

OK now you are ready for the trip to the store. Whether you have broken this process into three trips (one for each meal) or you are tackling all of the meals at once, use the Workbook pages at the back of the book for your food research.

Use the work pages to itemize the foods that sound good keeping track of the calorie, fat and sugar content. Once you have filled out the work pages you will use these pages to fill out the Meal Selection Final List that you can use when you create your shopping lists and menu guides.

If there are unhealthy foods that you just can not live without then don't live without them, just try to limit the serving sizes and try not to have them very often. Use them as a reward. If a diet plan were to tell me that I could never have French bread or Chocolate for the rest of my life, I could not stick to that diet.

Here are a couple of activities that may help with your diet:

- Try eating slower. You may find that you are actually overeating when you eat fast. By slowing down the consumption of your meals you will be able to recognize once you have eaten enough to be satisfied.

- Try chewing your food twice or three times as much as you would normally do. I read someplace that a person could lose weight by making sure that they chewed each bite at least 40 times. I know that it seems like a lot but it is worth a try.

- Try eating the less fattening items in your meal first. If you eat these slowly and chew them thoroughly you may become full prior to eating all of the higher calorie items.

- Take smaller portions to start out with. Sometimes I even take a small amount and put the rest back in the refrigerator. If I want more I can always reheat the food but most of the time I find the smaller portions to be fine. Have you ever noticed that frozen foods that are low calorie are usually very small portions compared to what you normally cook for your self? When I eat these dinners I am not left feeling hungry so I can only conclude that I usually take more food than I really need and because I was taught to finish all of the food on my plate, I feel guilty if I throw any away. Taking smaller portions and putting the rest away for another meal even stretches the food budget.

- Don't feel guilty about throwing food away. If you are full the worse thing you can do is to continue eating.

Exercises

I know for many, just the word exercise makes them gag. I know because I am one of those people.

That is because the word brings up pictures of sweat, unattractive clothing, treadmills and weight cages.

The truth about exercise is that it can be a lot more. It can be fun and it can be productive. In addition to toning your muscles, exercise can rev up your metabolism meaning that you burn more calories even when you are not exercising. This is great when you are on a diet because you will be able to eat more and still get the benefits of the diet.

I am going to start by listing some of my favorite exercises. Once you have reviewed my list you can go to the section in the back of the book entitled activity list (notice that I did not say exercise). When you fill out the activity list put down only activities that you like to do or at least activities that you can tolerate. I do not expect to see jogging around a track on the list unless you are training for some sort of race.

Once you have a list of your favorite activities then add a number from 1 to 10 (with 10 being the most strenuous and 1 being the least) to indicate the level of exercise that they provide. Dancing with grandchildren will most likely be a more strenuous activity than shopping unless you are doing one of my favorite the "Mall Walk".

Next add a few comments that list the obstacles to doing the activity. Dancing with grandchildren could be a problem if your grandchildren live on the other side of the country from you or if you have no grandchildren of your own (you may need to borrow some). Dog walking is not easy if you do not have a dog.

Following are some of my favorite exercises, none of which are done at a gym:

• Mall Walking

• Dog walking

• Bed exercises

- Dancing

- Swimming pool walking or swimming if you know how

- Gardening

- Hiking

- Shopping

- Bike riding

- Skating (ice and roller)

- Skiing (water and snow)

- All types of sports (not watching but playing)

- Playing with Grand Children

- Playing with puppies (one of my favorites)

- Sex

- Video games

Following are some of my less than favorite exercises also none of which are done at the gym.

- House work

- Leaf Raking

- Lawn Mowing

- Car Washing

- Tree Pruning

OK so I hate almost all exercises done on a track or at a gym. I like almost all forms of exercise out side of those.

Mall Walking

Mall Walking has always been one of my favorite exercises. The bigger the mall the better and more interesting it is for exercising.

I start at one end and walk the entire length without stopping at any of the shops. If I see something that interests me I will make a mental note that I want to return as soon as I am through with my exercise.

If you are really looking for an item on your shopping trip you may want to take a personal recorder of some type so that you can make note of the stores that you want to return to after you have finished with the exercise part of your shopping trip. This will work better than trying to remember all of the stores that you want to return to and will keep you from stopping because you are afraid that you will not remember.

I usually try to start at an end of the mall that has less of the shops that I like to frequent. By doing this I insure that I will get at least part of my exercise completed before I am tempted to end early and go shopping.

During my Mall Walk I also try to take the stairs instead of elevators or escalators. I park a good distance from the mall. I feel that this accomplishes two things: I get some exercise before I even reach the mall, and I save the closer parking spaces for people that need or want them more than I do.

Dog walking

I am not sure that you will want to get a dog just so that you can exercise but if you already have a dog it can be a wonderful bonding activity for you and your pet.

If, however, you are lonely and depressed getting a dog could be a good thing. You can gain a source of unconditional love, find a rewarding exercise and feel more protected or at least know that you will have some sort of warning if there is an intruder.

I used to own an Irish Wolfhound. We lived in a townhouse and the only real exercise that my dog would get is when I took her walking. She loved the walks and was so happy to see me with her leash that I never once had the heart to let her down.

I lost more weight in less time by walking that dog. Since I didn't ever weigh myself back then I know that I lost weight because a dropped multiple dress sizes. I also started feeling a lot better and had a lot more energy.

I know that I am very good at talking myself out of exercising when there isn't anyone or anything that is counting on me to go exercising. I felt awful any time I thought of skipping my walk with the dog because I knew how much she liked to go and how happy it made her when I took her.

I might add that I felt a lot safer while walking her than I would have had I been walking alone or with some friends. I know this because after a while I was no longer able to keep her at the townhouse and found it necessary to take her to my mother's house to live where there was an acreage for her to run around on. When I returned to the park where I used to take my dog for walks I was very uncomfortable. I discovered that there were a number of homeless people that lived in the park even though it was against the law. When I was walking the dog they stayed away from us, once I no longer had the dog with me they started harassing me in the same way that they bothered the other people who walked in the park and I felt uneasy enough with their harassment that I stopped going to that park altogether.

Bed exercises

Bed exercises are probably the easiest of the exercises to work into your schedule. I don't think that I know anyone who doesn't have a bed. If you are someone who lives in your car, try modifying the exercises to fit your surroundings.

I find myself unable to fall asleep many nights. I don't know if doing the exercises make me tired or if they just help to clear my mind but I can usually fall asleep soon after doing these exercises.

You can probably be more creative than I am. Following is a list of the exercises that I do in bed.

- Leg lifts

- Crunches

- Muscle Tightening

Everyone knows how to do the first two of the exercises. When I do the muscle tightening I just contract what ever muscle I am targeting as tight as I can and hold it for a while. Some times I will lay on my stomach and try to tighten my stomach muscles enough to lift my stomach off of the bed. I pretend that I am trying to touch my backbone with my stomach muscles. I also will lay on my back and tighten my butt muscles as tight as I can as if I was trying to lift something that was sitting on my stomach.

Dancing

Dancing is a wonderful exercise that you can do socially or you can do alone. It is one of those fun activities that can be done for hours without feeling as though you are exercising at all.

While I never had a significant other that liked to go dancing most of my dancing has been done alone. I find if I put on one of my favorite records (boy am I showing my age) I mean if I put on one of my favorite CDs, I can dance around for a long time as long as no one comes in and sees me. I don't like doing many exercises when anyone is watching.

If you have a small child, dancing with a child can be a lot of fun for both you and the child.

I have even gone to a country western bar in the past where they were giving free Line Dancing lessons. Many of the line dances do not require you to have a partner. Line dancing is a lot of fun and good exercise.

I have even paid for dance lessons. Taking dance lessons allows you to not only learn some interesting steps but you get to dance with someone who really knows how to do the dance and if it is one of the fast dances it can be a lot of exercise. Group dance lessons are usually less expensive and when I was taking the lessons there were a lot of single people who would show up for the lessons so that you did not need to bring your own partner to participate.

Swimming pool walking or swimming if you know how

This is another of my favorite exercises whenever I am brave enough to go into a cold pool. If you have a heater on your pool then I am jealous. If you don't you might want to think about getting one if this exercise works well for you.

Doing exercises in water is very easy on your joints. The cold water keeps you from sweating which is one of the things that can make exercise uncomfortable. You can make up silly games if you have someone else in the pool with you.

My son and I used to do all sort of silly races. Of course I usually got at least a half of the pool head start to make things fair. We would do hopping on one foot races or holding a basketball and kicking with your feet races just anything to bring a little competition and make the exercise more fun.

There is even a company that has a product called "The Endless Pool". This appears to be a very small pool with a water current generator. This pool provides you exercise when you swim against this current. I think this is a great idea and I hope sometime in the future to be able to purchase one of these pools to put in my house. I think this would be a wonderful exercise for just about any one at any age.

Gardening

I know it doesn't seem like gardening is an exercise. It is, however, if you are digging or walking up and down hills carrying fruit and vegetables.

My garden is built on a hillside and it produces a lot of food. I know from the feeling in my muscles after walking up and down the hill five or six times with buckets full of vegetables or fruit that I have gotten a lot of exercise. I know it even more when my muscles hurt for days afterwards.

If you don't have a hillside garden to work in, you are more than welcome to come work in mine.

OK, well seriously, you may have a friend who has a garden and needs help. You might be able to trade work for some the vegetable produce from the garden. I love the taste of vine ripened tomatoes, I hate most of the tomatoes that you find in the stores.

I might mention here that tomatoes are one of my favorite foods. I love tomato salads or eating cherry tomatoes right off of the vine. The reason that you will not find tomatoes on my list of snacks is that I seldom have tomatoes unless they come from a garden that either I have at my house or that my mother has at her house. I refuse to pay for tasteless tomatoes in a store. There truly is no substitute for vine ripened tomatoes.

Shopping

When I go shopping I park as far away from the store as I can without leaving the parking lot. This accomplishes two things. One: I get some extra exercise walking to the store and Two: It keeps my car door from being dinged since most everyone else is fighting for parking spots right in front of the store.

Depending on the type of shopping I am doing the process inside the store may be different. If I am shopping for food, I get out my grocery list, locate the produce on my list, pay for my items and then I leave. I try not to spend too much time inside a food store because the longer I walk around in the store the more bad foods jump into my shopping cart.

OK so if I am not going food shopping, I walk up and down all of the isles to see all of the items that they may have on sale and make sure that I have located the best of what ever I have come to the store to buy.

Once I have scoped out the store I then get the item that I came for and sometimes a few more items. I might note that I am really into Retail Therapy. I pay for the items and then I walk back to my car that is parked far, far away. If I have purchased a lot at a store that lacks shopping carts I get the additional exercise of carrying the shopping bags.

Many years ago when I was without a car I would walk to the store every day to buy the food for the next day. I would guess that the walk was about a mile one way. I could never buy enough for two days because I had to carry the bags home and one day of food was as heavy as I could carry that distance. Once I moved back with my family after having done this for three months I had dropped 2 dress sizes and had firmed up muscles that I didn't even know that I had.

Bike riding

Bike riding is an exercise that can even save money. If you live close enough to work it is a great method for commuting. You can also ride a bike to go shopping or just to ride.

Where I live there are some great bike trails and if you like communing with nature you can travel much longer distances than if you are hiking.

If you decide to get your exercise from biking you may need to brush up on the traffic laws. It is also advisable to get a checkup for your bike if it has been a while since you have ridden. If you don't want to be stranded you may want to consider buying a lock for your bike. My son had two bikes stolen, one from in front of a store and the other from his girlfriend's front steps. It can be a long walk home if the bike is suddenly missing.

Skating (ice and roller)

I haven't done either of these for a long time but when I used to go ice or roller skating it was a lot of fun and some good exercise. It is also a good way to get a lot of bruises.

Skiing (water and snow)

I am not good at either water or snow skiing and I have only done each of these activities once in my past. I know that there are many people that love both of these sports.

I have been told that cross country skiing is more exercise than downhill skiing. That might be different if you actually walked up the hill instead of riding the lift.

All types of sports (not watching but playing)

Sports participation is a subject that I know near to nothing about. Having been awkward as a child, I was nearly always chosen last in school for any types of sports. This experience was so demoralizing that I found myself avoiding playing sports my entire life.

I do know, however, from watching people playing sports and from talking to people who participate in sporting activities that most sports give you a lot of exercise. Even golf if you walk instead of using a golf cart is a lot of exercise. When you do something that you enjoy it will not feel as though you are exercising and you will be more apt to get more exercise out of the activity than you would if you were simply walking around a track.

Another good form of exercise and one that I have not done for many many years is Horse Back Riding. I know you are going to say that the horse is the one getting the exercise. When I used to ride, I owned the horse and I had it pastured on a 700+ acre ranch. I got a lot of exercise walking around in the pasture looking for the horse. Even if you don't have to go retrieve your horse the riding is still good exercise. When you ride a horse you are required to use muscles to balance yourself in ways that few of those muscles are used in normal daily living.

Playing with Grandchildren

Playing with grandchildren or playing with your own children can be a great form of exercise and entertainment. Once again, whenever you can get exercise that is enjoyable it will feel more like fun and less like a chore. Most exercise for exercise sake is not fun and feels more like a punishment for over eating. When an activity is not fun it is easier to make up excuses to get out of doing it and thus not getting the benefits that could be derived from exercise.

If you plan activities with your children or your grandchildren and you talk to them ahead of time, then you will be less apt to back out because they are counting on you.

Playing with puppies (one of my favorite exercises)

This is without a doubt one of my favorite exercises. I have an 11 month old Rat Terrier that thinks that any time I am out of bed that it is time to play. Actually he thinks it is playtime even when I am in bed.

His favorite game is try to catch the puppy when the puppy has something in his mouth that you don't want him to have. He loves to steal toilet paper and Kleenex and if you don't catch him he will shred and spread the paper all over the house.

He also likes to steal dollar bills out of a purse because depending on the denomination he gets a lot of attention when he plays keep away with that item.

Sex

I recommend this exercise only in committed relationships. This recommendation is not because I am old fashioned. Sex, as an exercise, has a lot of possible health and financial hazards. With all of the sexually transmitted diseases that exist, sex with casual partners is like playing Russian roulette with your life. Even if you don't get some untreatable disease you could find yourself financially ruined by an unwanted pregnancy.

That said, if you are going to have sex anyway you might as well get some exercise benefits from the activity. So as long as you are not just laying there it will be exercise and the more actively you participate (some people call this passion) the more exercise benefit you will get. You might not want to share with your partner that your new found passion and appreciation of sex is just so that you can get the benefits of the exercise that it provides. Let them think that you just find them irresistible.

Video Games

I know that this seems odd for an exercise buy my son assures me that there are games that have sensors that detect your movement. One of the games that gives a great deal of exercise is a dancing game that has a pad that you work on.

I plan to look into these soon. I think that they sound like fun.

Housework

Housework is exercise! If you have a two story home it is even more exercise. You could try putting on some of your favorite music and dance while you are doing the housework, this could make it more fun plus bumping up the benefits you get from the exercise because you put more effort into it.

No one will ever tell me that vigorous scrubbing of a floor is not more exercise than a light mopping. Even if the activity does not leave you breathless from exertion it does not mean that you have not gotten a good workout. Housework is usually a combination of Aerobic, Anaerobic and stretching. Anyone who thinks that they have not gotten a workout should take note of how their muscles feel in a couple of days.

A standup vacuum cleaner, a broom, or a mop can be very agile dance partners. Of course I would never do any of this if my husband or son were in the house to see me but in their absence I do a lot of silly things that I would not want on video tape.

Time Budgeting

I have found that a diet and exercise plan's success or failure hinges on one's ability to budget their time.

I am sure that you have all heard people say "Oh he is a morning person" or "She is a night owl".

Many people just do better when they start their day very early in the morning while others can't seem to get started until well into the day.

The time frame where you schedule your exercise routine within your day can also be a very personal preference. I know that I must schedule any exercise that I am going to do early in the morning, unless I am doing one of the aforementioned exercises that I find to be fun. I can do the "Mall Walk", Gardening, or playing with puppies almost anytime in the day and be successful at the activity.

No, I mean real exercising like the Treadmill, aerobics or weight lifting, these exercises require forethought, planning and travel. By this I mean that you do not usually do these types of exercises on a whim. You must dress for the occasion, few of us have the proper equipment at home so we must travel to the gym to do these exercises and we must plan to have enough time once we get to the gym to actually accomplish the planned exercise.

You will need to plan these exercise types at a time that works for your daily routine and energy level. While you may have most of your free time available in the evening, if you are physically drained from either stress or your type of work then this time period will not work for you. If however you have too much energy at night to make relaxing an option the evening may be just the perfect time for your exercise routine.

Helpful Tips

I have found a few helpful tips for sticking to a diet during some of the situations that used to ruin my own diets.

At the Casino or Bar:

If you are out on the town and your friends are drinking, you can order virgin drinks. With the calorie content of most alcoholic drinks being well over 100 calories I would hate to see you trash your diet for a drink that you probably don't even enjoy. I know that when I used to frequent social gatherings where alcohol was being served, I did not enjoy most of the drinks that were available and I certainly did not enjoy hanging over the toilet hours later sicker than a dog and swearing that I would never drink again. Most people drink just because every one else is doing it. The trick is to have as much fun socializing while consuming less calories.

One of my favorite drinks in these situations is a Virgin Mary. If I am hungry I will ask for one with extra olives, this will satisfy me enough that I can stay away from some of the higher calorie snacks that are available at parties. If I feel brave I will even order an extra spicy Virgin Mary. Be careful with this one because you never know how spicy "extra spicy" means to the bar tender. This drink has some added benefits in that they say that tomato juice a good source of vitamins and minerals.

When you are gambling a virgin drink can keep you sober so that you will not make as many stupid mistakes. My Virgin Mary with extra olives can keep me from needing to leave a machine to eat.

At a Birthday party, Baby Shower, Anniversary Party or any other celebration:

I know when I go to an event were they are celebrating and they are serving cake I feel as though I am saying that I am not happy for them if I do not eat some of the cake. This said, I could ask for a smaller piece of cake and avoid the outside edges of the cake where the calorie content with the added icing is much higher.

If you are in a position where the cake is self serve you can always take the smallest interior slice of cake, eat a few bites and then put it down someplace and forget where you left it. I know this sounds wasteful but I know from experience that most people will not eat or drink something that they have abandoned for a short period of time because they are not quite sure that it is theirs.

I have half full bottles of water left all over my property on hot days when I have outside help on work projects. I will take a couple of drinks from a newly opened water bottle put it down with all good intentions that I will return to finish it. When I do return, I am never quite sure that it is my water bottle so I leave it until my workers have left for the day and then I dump all of the left over water and throw away the bottles.

Lastly you can always take your cake, eat a few bites and wait until it is time to leave and throw the remaining cake away. I know from experience that throwing food away can make you feel very guilty. You may think of how lucky you are to have the food and that other less fortunate people in the world are starving as you contemplate whether or not to throw cake that could save their lives away. Trust me, no matter how hard you try, you will not save any starving people by gaining an extra pound yourself.

At the Office:

If your office work experience is anything like mine was, people are always making special treats and bringing them to work to share. You feel obligated to eat some of the treats even if you don't like them so that you do not hurt the feelings of the person that brought them.

Here again, moderation is the key. You don't have to eat an entire coffee cake to prove to your friend that you like her cooking. If the treats are not moving fast enough you could even volunteer to share some with a neighboring office. The trick is to eat only a little so that you can sound intelligent if you are asked how you like the treat, and remove the temptation as fast as possible. I know that where treats were left in my office I would go back for more not wanting my friend to feel that the treats were not enjoyed or appreciated.

On the Go:

When you are in a hurry and you stop to eat at a fast food restaurant, think about what you are ordering. While the main ingredients in a salad are very low in calories, as soon as you add the salad dressing, your salad may contain more calories than the dreaded HAMBURGER.

Just think about your selection. A small hamburger without cheese is certainly less damaging to your diet than a double cheese burger. Most people would be satisfied with far less food if they just stopped eating for a short period of time and waited to see if they felt full.

Always check the value meal menu. These entries are usually smaller than the regular sized dishes and may end up with only half the calorie content of the regular size. There is an added bonus to the value meals and that is that they cost less. So while you are protecting your waistline you may also be protecting your wallet by ordering from the value menu.

In real restaurants, always check the side dish menu. Cottage cheese or vegetable soup are always less damaging to a diet than a hamburger and French fries or a mega breakfast entry. This is also a good way to cut the cost of your meal in addition to cutting the calories in your meal.

One of the best ways to avoid calories when you are in a hurry to eat, is to carry low calorie satisfying snacks with you so that you can eat on the go and avoid stopping for food in the first place.

The Sandwich Alternative

I like sandwiches! Or to be more precise, I like the stuff that you put into sandwiches. Bread is usually the least tasty part of a sandwich and it is only there to hold the thing together.

Instead of having a sandwich, I take the normal ingredients for a sandwich and cut them into small pieces. I then take mustard or catsup and put a little on the plate with my cutup sandwich ingredients and use a fork to eat them like little shish kabobs. I really like doing this with the low calorie hotdogs. My plate will usually have cut up hotdog, tomato, onion, and dill pickle with a tablespoon or more of mustard. I might add that I also lose the lettuce which is pretty tasteless too.

Another possibility is roast beef, onion and tomato with a horseradish dip. You can also do smoked salmon, onion and tomato with a pureed horseradish and caper dip. As you can see the options are pretty much endless and oh so tasty.

Pre Made Ingredients

When I have the time, usually on the weekends, I will do a couple of hours of food preparation so that most of the work is already done when I make the weekday meals. My three favorite ingredients for making ahead are mushrooms and wine, onions and wine and onions and garlic. In the case of the mushrooms and onions in wine I just boil these after dicing or cutting to the desired size and I usually do this in the microwave. In the case of the garlic and onions, I will prepare them in one of two ways. I either dice the onions and garlic and then sauté them in olive oil or I puree the onions and garlic in a blender with olive oil and then cook them in the microwave. All of these prepared ingredients are subsequently placed in refrigerator containers for use during the week day meal prep. These ingredients allow me to make very tasty meals that would appear to have taken hours of cooking time in little or no time and my family is very impressed with the meals.

Water is your friend

While you are dieting or any other time for that matter, drink the recommended daily requirement of water. Your body will be at its healthiest when properly hydrated. Don't assume that just because you are consuming liquids that you have this requirement covered.

There are few things that you can add to your diet that are lower in calories than water. Drinking water with your meals can help you to feel full sooner. Adding some flavor to your water may help to replace your sugary sodas.

There are even some very effective diets that begin with three days of water fasting. I have yet to find any diet that required you to limit your intake of water.

Sometimes it helps if your daily menu is boring

I know I just went through a lot to convince you that your meals should be satisfying. When I am dieting I have always found that keeping my breakfast and lunch down to a few simple selections help me adhere to the diet.

Most days I have unsweetened shredded wheat with vanilla flavored soy milk for breakfast. On the days that I do not have the shredded wheat then I have an egg over easy on dry toast. I find that I get into a lot less trouble when I eat this way. I know how many calories these two meals contain and I know what amount of calories I have left for the rest of the day if I want to stick to a reduced calorie diet.

For lunch I usually have a low calorie meal that I heat in the microwave. These have the calories already calculated for me. On the days that I do not eat one of these meals I usually do a breadless sandwich. This can be either lunch meat rolled around a pickle, a tomato and an onion or it can be a low calorie hotdog cut in pieces that is eaten by spearing tomato, pickle and onion prior to spearing the last ingredient which is the hotdog and then dipping it in mustard.

Snack Selection Work Pages

Snack Selection	Calories	Fat Content	Sugar	Serving Size
_____	_____	_____	_____	_____
_____	_____	_____	_____	_____
_____	_____	_____	_____	_____
_____	_____	_____	_____	_____
_____	_____	_____	_____	_____
_____	_____	_____	_____	_____
_____	_____	_____	_____	_____
_____	_____	_____	_____	_____
_____	_____	_____	_____	_____
_____	_____	_____	_____	_____
_____	_____	_____	_____	_____
_____	_____	_____	_____	_____
_____	_____	_____	_____	_____
_____	_____	_____	_____	_____
_____	_____	_____	_____	_____
_____	_____	_____	_____	_____
_____	_____	_____	_____	_____
_____	_____	_____	_____	_____
_____	_____	_____	_____	_____
_____	_____	_____	_____	_____
_____	_____	_____	_____	_____
_____	_____	_____	_____	_____
_____	_____	_____	_____	_____

Snack Selection	Calories	Fat Content	Sugar	Serving Size
_____	_____	_____	____	_____
_____	_____	_____	____	_____
_____	_____	_____	____	_____
_____	_____	_____	____	_____
_____	_____	_____	____	_____
_____	_____	_____	____	_____
_____	_____	_____	____	_____
_____	_____	_____	____	_____
_____	_____	_____	____	_____
_____	_____	_____	____	_____
_____	_____	_____	____	_____
_____	_____	_____	____	_____
_____	_____	_____	____	_____
_____	_____	_____	____	_____
_____	_____	_____	____	_____
_____	_____	_____	____	_____
_____	_____	_____	____	_____
_____	_____	_____	____	_____
_____	_____	_____	____	_____
_____	_____	_____	____	_____
_____	_____	_____	____	_____
_____	_____	_____	____	_____
_____	_____	_____	____	_____
_____	_____	_____	____	_____
_____	_____	_____	____	_____
_____	_____	_____	____	_____
_____	_____	_____	____	_____

Snack Selection	Calories	Fat Content	Sugar	Serving Size

Snack Selection	Calories	Fat Content	Sugar	Serving Size
_____	_____	_____	_____	_____
_____	_____	_____	_____	_____
_____	_____	_____	_____	_____
_____	_____	_____	_____	_____
_____	_____	_____	_____	_____
_____	_____	_____	_____	_____
_____	_____	_____	_____	_____
_____	_____	_____	_____	_____
_____	_____	_____	_____	_____
_____	_____	_____	_____	_____
_____	_____	_____	_____	_____
_____	_____	_____	_____	_____
_____	_____	_____	_____	_____
_____	_____	_____	_____	_____
_____	_____	_____	_____	_____
_____	_____	_____	_____	_____
_____	_____	_____	_____	_____
_____	_____	_____	_____	_____
_____	_____	_____	_____	_____
_____	_____	_____	_____	_____
_____	_____	_____	_____	_____
_____	_____	_____	_____	_____
_____	_____	_____	_____	_____
_____	_____	_____	_____	_____
_____	_____	_____	_____	_____
_____	_____	_____	_____	_____
_____	_____	_____	_____	_____
_____	_____	_____	_____	_____
_____	_____	_____	_____	_____

Snack Selection	Calories	Fat Content	Sugar	Serving Size

Food Selection Work Pages

Food Selection	Calories	Fat Content	Sugar	Serving Size
_____	_____	_____	_____	_____
_____	_____	_____	_____	_____
_____	_____	_____	_____	_____
_____	_____	_____	_____	_____
_____	_____	_____	_____	_____
_____	_____	_____	_____	_____
_____	_____	_____	_____	_____
_____	_____	_____	_____	_____
_____	_____	_____	_____	_____
_____	_____	_____	_____	_____
_____	_____	_____	_____	_____
_____	_____	_____	_____	_____
_____	_____	_____	_____	_____
_____	_____	_____	_____	_____
_____	_____	_____	_____	_____
_____	_____	_____	_____	_____
_____	_____	_____	_____	_____
_____	_____	_____	_____	_____
_____	_____	_____	_____	_____
_____	_____	_____	_____	_____
_____	_____	_____	_____	_____
_____	_____	_____	_____	_____
_____	_____	_____	_____	_____
_____	_____	_____	_____	_____

Food Selection	Calories	Fat Content	Sugar	Serving Size

Food Selection	Calories	Fat Content	Sugar	Serving Size
————————	————	————	———	—————
————————	————	————	———	—————
————————	————	————	———	—————
————————	————	————	———	—————
————————	————	————	———	—————
————————	————	————	———	—————
————————	————	————	———	—————
————————	————	————	———	—————
————————	————	————	———	—————
————————	————	————	———	—————
————————	————	————	———	—————
————————	————	————	———	—————
————————	————	————	———	—————
————————	————	————	———	—————
————————	————	————	———	—————
————————	————	————	———	—————
————————	————	————	———	—————
————————	————	————	———	—————
————————	————	————	———	—————
————————	————	————	———	—————
————————	————	————	———	—————
————————	————	————	———	—————
————————	————	————	———	—————
————————	————	————	———	—————
————————	————	————	———	—————
————————	————	————	———	—————
————————	————	————	———	—————

Food Selection	Calories	Fat Content	Sugar	Serving Size
_____	_____	_____	_____	_____
_____	_____	_____	_____	_____
_____	_____	_____	_____	_____
_____	_____	_____	_____	_____
_____	_____	_____	_____	_____
_____	_____	_____	_____	_____
_____	_____	_____	_____	_____
_____	_____	_____	_____	_____
_____	_____	_____	_____	_____
_____	_____	_____	_____	_____
_____	_____	_____	_____	_____
_____	_____	_____	_____	_____
_____	_____	_____	_____	_____
_____	_____	_____	_____	_____
_____	_____	_____	_____	_____
_____	_____	_____	_____	_____
_____	_____	_____	_____	_____
_____	_____	_____	_____	_____
_____	_____	_____	_____	_____
_____	_____	_____	_____	_____
_____	_____	_____	_____	_____
_____	_____	_____	_____	_____
_____	_____	_____	_____	_____
_____	_____	_____	_____	_____
_____	_____	_____	_____	_____
_____	_____	_____	_____	_____
_____	_____	_____	_____	_____

Food Selection	Calories	Fat Content	Sugar	Serving Size
_____	_____	_____	_____	_____
_____	_____	_____	_____	_____
_____	_____	_____	_____	_____
_____	_____	_____	_____	_____
_____	_____	_____	_____	_____
_____	_____	_____	_____	_____
_____	_____	_____	_____	_____
_____	_____	_____	_____	_____
_____	_____	_____	_____	_____
_____	_____	_____	_____	_____
_____	_____	_____	_____	_____
_____	_____	_____	_____	_____
_____	_____	_____	_____	_____
_____	_____	_____	_____	_____
_____	_____	_____	_____	_____
_____	_____	_____	_____	_____
_____	_____	_____	_____	_____
_____	_____	_____	_____	_____
_____	_____	_____	_____	_____
_____	_____	_____	_____	_____
_____	_____	_____	_____	_____
_____	_____	_____	_____	_____
_____	_____	_____	_____	_____
_____	_____	_____	_____	_____
_____	_____	_____	_____	_____
_____	_____	_____	_____	_____
_____	_____	_____	_____	_____

Snack Selection Final list

Snack Selection	Calories	Fat Content	Sugar	Serving Size
_____	_____	_____	_____	_____
_____	_____	_____	_____	_____
_____	_____	_____	_____	_____
_____	_____	_____	_____	_____
_____	_____	_____	_____	_____
_____	_____	_____	_____	_____
_____	_____	_____	_____	_____
_____	_____	_____	_____	_____
_____	_____	_____	_____	_____
_____	_____	_____	_____	_____
_____	_____	_____	_____	_____
_____	_____	_____	_____	_____
_____	_____	_____	_____	_____
_____	_____	_____	_____	_____
_____	_____	_____	_____	_____
_____	_____	_____	_____	_____
_____	_____	_____	_____	_____
_____	_____	_____	_____	_____
_____	_____	_____	_____	_____
_____	_____	_____	_____	_____
_____	_____	_____	_____	_____
_____	_____	_____	_____	_____
_____	_____	_____	_____	_____
_____	_____	_____	_____	_____

Food Selection Final list

Food Selection	Calories	Fat Content	Sugar	Serving Size
_____	_____	_____	_____	_____
_____	_____	_____	_____	_____
_____	_____	_____	_____	_____
_____	_____	_____	_____	_____
_____	_____	_____	_____	_____
_____	_____	_____	_____	_____
_____	_____	_____	_____	_____
_____	_____	_____	_____	_____
_____	_____	_____	_____	_____
_____	_____	_____	_____	_____
_____	_____	_____	_____	_____
_____	_____	_____	_____	_____
_____	_____	_____	_____	_____
_____	_____	_____	_____	_____
_____	_____	_____	_____	_____
_____	_____	_____	_____	_____
_____	_____	_____	_____	_____
_____	_____	_____	_____	_____
_____	_____	_____	_____	_____
_____	_____	_____	_____	_____
_____	_____	_____	_____	_____
_____	_____	_____	_____	_____
_____	_____	_____	_____	_____
_____	_____	_____	_____	_____

Food Selection	Calories	Fat Content	Sugar	Serving Size
_____	_____	_____	_____	_____
_____	_____	_____	_____	_____
_____	_____	_____	_____	_____
_____	_____	_____	_____	_____
_____	_____	_____	_____	_____
_____	_____	_____	_____	_____
_____	_____	_____	_____	_____
_____	_____	_____	_____	_____
_____	_____	_____	_____	_____
_____	_____	_____	_____	_____
_____	_____	_____	_____	_____
_____	_____	_____	_____	_____
_____	_____	_____	_____	_____
_____	_____	_____	_____	_____
_____	_____	_____	_____	_____
_____	_____	_____	_____	_____
_____	_____	_____	_____	_____
_____	_____	_____	_____	_____
_____	_____	_____	_____	_____
_____	_____	_____	_____	_____
_____	_____	_____	_____	_____
_____	_____	_____	_____	_____
_____	_____	_____	_____	_____
_____	_____	_____	_____	_____
_____	_____	_____	_____	_____
_____	_____	_____	_____	_____
_____	_____	_____	_____	_____
_____	_____	_____	_____	_____

Food Selection	Calories	Fat Content	Sugar	Serving Size
_____	_____	_____	_____	_____
_____	_____	_____	_____	_____
_____	_____	_____	_____	_____
_____	_____	_____	_____	_____
_____	_____	_____	_____	_____
_____	_____	_____	_____	_____
_____	_____	_____	_____	_____
_____	_____	_____	_____	_____
_____	_____	_____	_____	_____
_____	_____	_____	_____	_____
_____	_____	_____	_____	_____
_____	_____	_____	_____	_____
_____	_____	_____	_____	_____
_____	_____	_____	_____	_____
_____	_____	_____	_____	_____
_____	_____	_____	_____	_____
_____	_____	_____	_____	_____
_____	_____	_____	_____	_____
_____	_____	_____	_____	_____
_____	_____	_____	_____	_____
_____	_____	_____	_____	_____
_____	_____	_____	_____	_____
_____	_____	_____	_____	_____
_____	_____	_____	_____	_____
_____	_____	_____	_____	_____
_____	_____	_____	_____	_____

Menu Work Pages

Breakfast Day 1

Item	Calories
_____	_____
_____	_____
_____	_____
_____	_____
Total	_____

Lunch Day 1

Item	Calories
_____	_____
_____	_____
_____	_____
_____	_____
Total	_____

Dinner Day 1

Item	Calories
_____	_____
_____	_____
_____	_____
_____	_____
_____	_____
Total	_____
Daily Meal Total	_____

Snacks Day 1

Mid Morning

Item	Calories
_____	_____
_____	_____
_____	_____

Afternoon

Item	Calories
_____	_____
_____	_____
_____	_____

Evening

Item	Calories
_____	_____
_____	_____
_____	_____

Total Snacks	_____
Total for Day	_____

Breakfast Day 2

Item   Calories

_____   _____

_____   _____

_____   _____

_____   _____

Total   _____

Lunch Day 2

Item   Calories

_____   _____

_____   _____

_____   _____

_____   _____

Total   _____

Dinner Day 2

Item   Calories

_____   _____

_____   _____

_____   _____

_____   _____

_____   _____

Total   _____

Daily Meal Total   _____

Snacks Day 2

Mid Morning

Item   Calories

_____   _____

_____   _____

_____   _____

Afternoon

Item   Calories

_____   _____

_____   _____

_____   _____

Evening

Item   Calories

_____   _____

_____   _____

_____   _____

Total Snacks   _____

Total for Day   _____

Breakfast Day 3

Item   Calories

_____   _____

_____   _____

_____   _____

_____   _____

Total   _____

Lunch Day 3

Item   Calories

_____   _____

_____   _____

_____   _____

_____   _____

Total   _____

Dinner Day 3

Item   Calories

_____   _____

_____   _____

_____   _____

_____   _____

_____   _____

Total   _____

Daily Meal Total   _____

Snacks Day 3

Mid Morning

Item	Calories
_____	_____
_____	_____
_____	_____

Afternoon

Item	Calories
_____	_____
_____	_____
_____	_____

Evening

Item	Calories
_____	_____
_____	_____
_____	_____

Total Snacks   _____

Total for Day   _____

Activity list

Activity	Level	Comments
_____	____	_____
_____	____	_____
_____	____	_____
_____	____	_____
_____	____	_____
_____	____	_____
_____	____	_____
_____	____	_____
_____	____	_____
_____	____	_____
_____	____	_____
_____	____	_____
_____	____	_____
_____	____	_____
_____	____	_____
_____	____	_____
_____	____	_____
_____	____	_____
_____	____	_____
_____	____	_____
_____	____	_____
_____	____	_____
_____	____	_____

Activity	Level	Comments
_____	____	_____
_____	____	_____
_____	____	_____
_____	____	_____
_____	____	_____
_____	____	_____
_____	____	_____
_____	____	_____
_____	____	_____
_____	____	_____
_____	____	_____
_____	____	_____
_____	____	_____
_____	____	_____
_____	____	_____
_____	____	_____
_____	____	_____
_____	____	_____
_____	____	_____
_____	____	_____
_____	____	_____
_____	____	_____
_____	____	_____
_____	____	_____
_____	____	_____
_____	____	_____

Activity	Level	Comments
_____	___	_____
_____	___	_____
_____	___	_____
_____	___	_____
_____	___	_____
_____	___	_____
_____	___	_____
_____	___	_____
_____	___	_____
_____	___	_____
_____	___	_____
_____	___	_____
_____	___	_____
_____	___	_____
_____	___	_____
_____	___	_____
_____	___	_____
_____	___	_____
_____	___	_____
_____	___	_____
_____	___	_____
_____	___	_____
_____	___	_____
_____	___	_____
_____	___	_____
_____	___	_____
_____	___	_____

Activity	Level	Comments
_____	____	_____
_____	____	_____
_____	____	_____
_____	____	_____
_____	____	_____
_____	____	_____
_____	____	_____
_____	____	_____
_____	____	_____
_____	____	_____
_____	____	_____
_____	____	_____
_____	____	_____
_____	____	_____
_____	____	_____
_____	____	_____
_____	____	_____
_____	____	_____
_____	____	_____
_____	____	_____
_____	____	_____
_____	____	_____
_____	____	_____
_____	____	_____

978-0-595-48459-1
0-595-48459-X